Alkaline Ketogenic Juicing

Nutrient-Packed, Alkaline-Keto Juice Recipes for Balance, Energy, Holistic Health, and Natural Weight Loss

I0222507

By Elena Garcia

Copyright Elena Garcia © 2019

ISBN: 978-1-913517-02-1

Disclaimer

A physician has not written the information in this book. It is advisable that you visit a qualified dietician so that you can obtain a highly personalized treatment for your case, especially if you want to lose weight effectively. This book is for informational and educational purposes only and is not intended for medical purposes. Please consult your physician before making any drastic changes to your diet.

All information in this book has been carefully researched and checked for factual accuracy. However, the author and publishers

Contents

Introduction

Thank You for purchasing this book.

It means you are very serious about your health and wellbeing.

Whether your goal is to lose weight, enjoy more energy, or learn a few delicious healing juicing recipes- you have come to the right place. With this guide, you will learn the art of juicing the right way, the way that is good for you and supports your health and weight loss goals.

This recipe book is a practical guide designed for busy people who value their health and wellbeing. Alkaline Ketogenic juicing is super healthy, and it's compatible with low or no sugar diets as well as super low carb diets.

Enriching your diet with alkaline keto juice can help you:

1. Eliminate sugar cravings.
2. Start losing weight naturally.
3. Enjoy more energy and vibrant health.
4. Help your body heal naturally by giving it a myriad of nutrients to help it get back in balance it deserves.

This guide is NOT designed as a juice fast.

We recommend you follow a balanced, clean food diet with enough calories to meet your nutritional needs (you can check out the first book in the series called Alkaline Ketogenic Mix to learn delicious clean food, alkaline keto recipes you will never get bored with).

Then, add healthy alkaline keto juice on top of that, and you will be amazed by the results.

Unstoppable energy, healthy glow, feeling amazing. Everyone around you will want to know your secret. Not to mention feeling confident about your transformation and knowing you are treating your body with the respect it deserves!

To make it as doable and straightforward as possible:

1. We will cover the main differences between juicing and smoothies, and why juicing might be more helpful to help you reach some of your health, wellness, and fitness goals much faster.

2. Then, we will move onto the alkaline-keto shopping lists- so that you know what ingredients you need to focus on.

You can even start taking action right away, as you are reading this book. The ingredients are inexpensive and easy to find.

3. Then, I will guide you through straightforward explanations of the alkaline and keto diets, and how these two can be combined as well as the fantastic health and wellness benefits, you can experience by enriching your diet with nutrient-packed, low-carb, low-sugar alkaline keto juices.

4. Finally, I'll introduce you to my favorite alkaline-keto juicing recipes.

Juicing vs. Smoothies?

What I really like about alkaline-keto juices is that unlike traditional fruit juices or processed juices, they don't use any high sugar fruit. Healthy, balanced juicing must be done the right way.

Unfortunately, many people miss that point. It's not their fault at all. There is just so much misinformation out there.

You see, juicing is an incredible way to boost your energy levels. When you juice, you extract pure juice, and there is no fiber, and so that allows your digestive system to rest. All the nutrients get easily absorbed into your system, and your body doesn't need to do any "extra hours" to digest it. Hence the almost instant energy boost and natural high.

Since there is nothing to digest and with juicing you give your body a ton of nutrients, you naturally start experiencing more energy. However, juicing must be done the right way. Otherwise, you can really mess up your health goals. For example, if you juice fruit that is high in sugar, you will only cause havoc in your body. With no fiber, it's pure sugar that gets absorbed to your system to start causing imbalance.

Fruit is OK, as a part of a balanced, clean food diet, but juicing fruit that is high in sugar is not good for you. That is why I am a fan of alkaline keto style of juicing. With this method of juicing, you focus on low-sugar or no sugar ingredients. Veggies and fruit that are low in sugar.

These are examples of fruits that are low in sugar: lemons, limes, grapefruits, tomatoes, pomegranates (more in the next section where we will scrutinize all the food lists).

Because of their low sugar and high mineral content, they are considered alkaline-forming fruits. Alkaline diet doesn't like sugar (keto diet is very similar in this regard). If you are new to the alkaline and keto diets, that is one of the most important lessons, and it can really help you revolutionize your health.

Years ago, I was very desperate to lose weight, always signing up for all kinds of fads. I also tried juicing, but it didn't work for me, because I wasn't taught to do it the right way.

First of all, juicing all the fancy fruit was getting very expensive. And, I couldn't lose weight, and my health and energy levels were deteriorating because of all the sweet sugar-packed fruit juice I was drinking.

That is why I am so passionate about writing this book. I want to show you the right way, the balanced approach. And I will mention it again, especially for you young females out there- please eat enough and don't starve yourself with juices. The recipes in this book are not a meal replacement. Instead, use it as a delicious and nutritious drink to sip on during the day, in between your meals.

Ok, so now let's compare juicing to smoothies. As you already know, juices extract the healing elixirs while getting rid of the pulp. It works great if you need a quick, natural energy boost while giving your digestive system a rest. It also works great for people who, for whatever health reason, can't tolerate too much fiber in their food. For example, my mom, even though she likes smoothies, can't have too much of them because of her digestive issues. That is why she's more focused on juicing.

Personally, I love both. I am also a big fan of healthy smoothies. To learn more about the Alkaline Keto smoothies, I recommend you read the second book in the Alkaline Keto Diet series: Alkaline Ketogenic Smoothies.
Ok, now that I have praised juicing and got you all excited (that was good news actually), I also have some bad news for you...

Well, it's not really that bad...as they say no pain no gain, right?

Ok, so here it is...making juices is a bit more time-consuming than blending smoothies. And it may take a bit more time to clean up.

My recommendation is to schedule your juicing time, for example, 2-3 times a week. Be sure to "batch-juice." That way, one juicing session can cover your juicing for the following day as well. You can store your fresh juice in a fridge, for no more than 24 hours.

Also, as you keep juicing more and more, you will get faster and faster. Trust me on that one! You will soon be a juicing expert (well, maybe you already are, who knows?).

For my smoothies, I use Vitamix Blender (but any blender will do as long as it works). For juicing, I use another tool, a fantastic juicer called Omega juicer. I love their brand. When choosing a juicer, be sure to use a cold press juicer that can also handle juicing a ton of greens.

You can learn more about my juicing recommendations and tools to help you on your juicing journey on my website:

www.YourWellnessBooks.com/resources

Finally, the recipes, as well as "nutritional philosophies" contained in this book, are very flexible and open-minded. Anyone can benefit from them; they are not only for people who follow alkaline or keto diets. So, whether you are alkaline keto full-time, or merely part-time (you are looking for easy tips and recipes to improve your health), you have come to the right place! Everyone can benefit from the power of alkaline keto juicing.

The moment you decide to focus on the abundance of healthy foods, you will automatically start craving all the good stuff.

So, without any further ado, let's do this. I am so excited for You!

Alkaline Keto Juices- Food Lists

Recommended Alkaline Keto Fruit

Both alkaline, as well as ketogenic diets, encourage you to stay away from sugar, including fruit that is high in sugar.

However, low-sugar fruits are allowed, and there are many ways to make them taste delicious (the recipes will show you how):

Alkaline Keto Approved Fruits:

- Limes
- Lemons
- Grapefruits
- Avocado (yes, it's a fruit)
- Tomato (yea, it's a fruit)
- Pomegranate

The following fruit is allowed occasionally, in small amounts, to flavor, infuse, or garnish:

- Green apple (sparingly)
- Orange (also sparingly)

Recommended Alkaline Keto Greens

Greens are very good for you, and if used correctly, they will taste really nice in your juices. Don't worry if you have never made any green juice before, or are not too sure how it will taste. The recipes contained in this book got you covered.

While it may be tough to eat 4 cucumbers, 2 cups of spinach, 3 zucchini's with 3 red bell peppers and a bunch of kale, it's easy to drink their nutrients. Adding some greens to your salads and smoothies is already a significant step forward. But...juicing greens is a real game changer! Trust me on that one.

All leafy greens are super alkaline and also compatible with keto diets:

- Spinach
- Kale
- Microgreens
- Swiss Chard
- Arugula
- Endive
- Romaine Lettuce

+ other fresh leafy greens and greens as well as:

- Parsley
- Mint
- Cilantro

I prefer fresh greens to green powders…but…whenever I go traveling, or I am really pressed for time, I use a delicious green powder blend called Organifi.

I also like to add it to my recipes as it makes my juices taste really nice while adding a ton of superfoods at the same time.

You can learn more about it and how I use it with my recipes on my website (treat it as an additional recommendation):

www.yourwellnessbooks.com/resources

Alkaline Keto Friendly Vegetables

All fresh veggies are considered alkaline, and most of them are also keto because they are low in carbs and low in sugar. The juice recipes from this book also call for good fats (more on the good fats later) to create alkaline keto balance and use fats for energy, instead of carbs.

So, these are the best alkaline – keto veggies to use in your juices:

- Red bell pepper
- Green bell pepper
- Yellow bell pepper
- Zucchini
- Broccoli
- Asparagus
- Colliflower
- Garlic
- Cucumbers
- Radishes

Alkaline Keto Spices & Herbs for Your Juices

The following herbs and spices will make your juices taste delicious.
They are also full of anti-inflammatory properties.

Again, since there are no sugars and no nasty carbs, the following
herbs and spices are both alkaline and keto friendly.

- Cinnamon
- Himalaya Salt
- Curry
- Red Chili Powder
- Cumin
- Nutmeg
- Italian spices
- Oregano
- Rosemary
- Lavender
- Mint
- Chamomile
- Fennel
- Cilantro
- Moringa

Alkaline Keto Sweeteners and Supplements (Optional)

Stevia (very helpful if you want to make a sweet juice without using sugar or sugar-containing foods or supplements)

- Green Powders, like Organifi
- Spirulina
- Chorella
- Matcha
- Moringa Powder
- Maca Powder
- Ashwagandha Powder

Again, these are all optional. However, if you are interested in learning more, please visit our private website where I share more complimentary info with my readers. I have listed my favorite brands, green powders, and other health supplements to help you save your time on research:

www.YourWellnessBooks.com/resources

Alkaline Keto Fats

Plant-Based

(these are both alkaline and keto friendly)

- Olive oil (organic, cold-pressed)
- Avocado oil
- Hemp oil
- Flaxseed oil
- Coconut oil
- Sesame oil

(please note, there is no need to purchase all of them, one, or two is enough; my two favorites are coconut oil and olive oil)

Animal Based

(these are more keto than alkaline because the alkaline diet prefers plant-based products. However, they are OK to use on a balanced diet full of greens and veggies)

- Organic butter
- Fish oil

Still, for the purpose of this book, we will be focusing mostly on plant-based fats because they work much better for juicing recipes. However, other books in this series:

Book 1 – Alkaline Ketogenic Mix **&**

Book 2 – Alkaline Ketogenic Smoothies

Also, call for animal fats in some recipes.

Alkaline Keto Friendly Milk & Other Liquids to Use in Your Juices

While these are not the main ingredients, they do work really well for some recipes. For example, some juicing recipes may taste way too intense, and so it makes sense to mix them with some alkaline-keto friendly liquids. Also, mixing your juices with other alkaline-keto friendly liquids will make your juicing habits less expensive.

Plant-Based

(these are both alkaline and keto friendly)

- Almond milk
- Coconut milk
- Hazelnut milk
- Coconut water
- Herbal infusions

- Organic Apple Cider Vinegar

+ coffee and caffeine, in moderation (for example, you can combine your juice with a little bit of green tea or red tea).

If you have any questions about the food lists for alkaline keto juices, please email me:

info@yourwellnessbooks.com

You can also sign up for our free newsletter at:

www.yourwellnessbooks.com/email-newsletter

and then reply to my first email and say hi.

Please note, the lists I have shared are essential food lists to make alkaline keto friendly juices because I want to keep it as simple as possible.

But they are not set in stone. I am always happy to answer your questions regarding the ingredients you want to use in your juices. Now, let's move on to the next part!

Why Alkaline Ketogenic Juices? How Can They Help You?

The problem is that most people eat way too many carbs and sugars. The temptations are everywhere, I know! To make it even worse, we eat processed carbs and sugars (pasta, candy, cakes, etc.). Most people find it hard to start their day without carbs and sugar.

Luckily, once you get into the alkaline ketogenic lifestyle, through adding some delicious low-carb, low sugar, high-fat juices into your diet, you will be able to experience a whole range of health and wellness benefits as well as possible prevention of many diseases.

Low carb, low sugar diets are proven to:

-manage your sugar levels, prevent diabetes

-normalize your hormones and auto-immune system

-improve your neurological health

-have even been used in clinical settings to prevent Alzheimer's, epilepsies, type 3 diabetes

Alkaline-Keto juicing is the healthiest method of juicing- you are giving your body an instant injection of nutrients. That allows you to enjoy more energy naturally, you no longer crave carbohydrates and sugars.

Most sugar cravings we experience happen because our body is not feeling nourished...It's calling for help- *please, feed me! I am still hungry. Yes, I know, you fed me with pizza, ice cream, and a milkshake and you have been drinking coffee all day. But I am still tired. Can you please feed me with something so that I can actually do my job? My job is to keep you healthy. My job is to burn fat. My job is to make you look and feel amazing. Just, please! Feed me with something that will help me, will ya?*

Ok, rant finished 😊

Here are other benefits of aligning your dietary choices with an alkaline ketogenic-friendly way:
-you will experience reduced hunger and reduced cravings
-you will be burning fat and reducing carbs and so normalizing your insulin levels
-you will protect your heart while raising the good cholesterol
-you will enjoy the anti-age benefits, as keto foods promote longevity and vitality (while nobody ever promised us we will live forever, by making a decision to stay healthy, we make sure that the time we are here on earth, we feel good and are vibrant).

Your transformation starts right here, right now.

Alkaline Keto juices are one of the best and easiest tools to help you get started, even if you are new to living a healthy lifestyle.

Now, let's have a look at:

1. What the keto diet actually is.
2. What the alkaline diet is.
3. How these two can be successfully combined for optimal benefits while respecting your nutritional lifestyle choices and preferences.

The goal of this book is simple- I don't want to "push" any specific kind of a diet bandwagon or make you feel bad for eating a certain way.

Making people feel bad or fear-based marketing tactics never lead to any long-term transformation. Unfortunately, this is how most of the nutrition- health and fitness industry operates- fear-based marketing tactics and making people feel bad.

Instead, I want to inspire you and give you simple, healthy, and delicious tools (alkaline ketogenic juices) to help you get closer to your health, wellness, and fitness goals every day.

How about setting one simple goal, to begin with? Drink 1 alkaline ketogenic juice a day? Take meaningful I and inspired action from a place of curiosity and empowerment, not fear.

Forget about perfection and focus on progress...

We are very, very close to help you get started. In fact, if you have already read my book *Alkaline Ketogenic Mix,* or *Alkaline Diet for Weight Loss and Wellness,* or *Alkaline Paleo Mix,* feel free to skip the following section and dive right into the recipes.

What really matters here is practice. But a little bit of inspiring information and learning more about our amazing bodies can also help.

So...

What Is the Keto Diet?

The simplest definition is:

The ketogenic diet is a diet low in carbs and high in healthy fats.

It encourages to massively reduce the carbohydrate intake and replace it with good, healthy fats (more on healthy vs. unhealthy fats later). This cutback in carbs puts your body into a metabolic state called ketosis.

When in ketosis, your body becomes super-efficient at burning fat for energy. A ketogenic diet can also help reduce blood sugar and insulin levels.

The fact is that we are designed to have periods where we "fast from carbs" and when our glucose levels are depleted.

Then, we start using our body very cleverly, using ketones for fuel. Ketones are the result of our body burning fat for food. The liver converts body fats and ingested fats into ketones.

Transition your diet into a more keto-friendly diet, it's straightforward. It means fewer sugars and carbs and more good fats while eating well!

Following this simple rule (even without going keto full-time) will help you transform your health. It will also help you lose weight naturally if you stay committed to it.

You will no longer be hooked on all those "crappy carbs" and with the new "keto energy" you will feel much more motivated to work out and be more active.

So, here's what the ketogenic diet consists of:

-75%- 80% fat (don't worry, it's all good fat and will not make you fat).

-5-15% healthy, clean protein

-5% good, unprocessed carbs (yea, you can still eat some carbs and the carbs we will be focusing on, will be healthy unprocessed no sugar carbs so no worries, there is no starvation involved here).

What Is the Alkaline Diet?

"Going green" is the way to describe an alkaline diet and lifestyle because the focus is on green vegetables in general, as they are the most alkaline food you can ingest.

The benefits of the alkaline diet are numerous. Let us name a few:

WEIGHT LOSS

An alkaline diet will assist you in losing weight. One way that it does this is obvious. The foods you will be eating are very healthy, rich in minerals and low calorie in general.

You will also be reducing the amount of acid in your body. The body stores fat to protect itself from an abundance of acid. It is a self-preservation method. This is part of the reason why people who exercise a lot and drink an excess of caffeine cannot seem to lose those extra pounds. Their bodies are clinging to that fat to minimize the effects of all of the acid in their systems. Caffeine is really acid-forming, and it's not the most sustainable source of energy. That is why we recommend you drink it in moderation, for your own occasional enjoyment rather than a source of energy you depend on.

Another benefit of an alkaline lifestyle regarding weight loss is that alkaline systems have more oxygen in their cells. Oxygen is a very essential part of eliminating fat cells from the body. The more oxygen in your system, the more efficient your metabolism will be.

ENERGY

Going green does not only give you energy for the apparent reason that you are eating many more healthy, energizing vitamins. You are negating the acid-induced lethargy that is brought on by an unhealthy acid-forming diet.

Not only do our bodies need an abundance of oxygen to lose weight, but we also need oxygen in our cells to energize us. The lack of oxygen in our cells causes fatigue. No, it is not just because you worked too late or partied to hard the night before. It is internal. If your cells are trying to function in a highly acidic environment, they will not be able to transfer oxygen efficiently; leading of course to exhaustion.

Cells in the body also make something that is called adenosine triphosphate (ATP). If your system is very acidic, it harms the ability of your cells to produce it. In the scientific world, it is known as the "energy currency of life." The ATP molecule contains the energy that we need to accomplish most things that we do (both internally and externally).

BODILY FUNCTIONS

Another benefit of the alkaline lifestyle is that your body will be able to function at an optimum level instead of being inhibited by acids:

- Your heartbeat is thrown off by acidic wastes in the body. The stomach suffers greatly from over-acidity.
- The liver's job is to get rid of acid toxins, but also to produce alkaline enzymes. By simply reducing your acid intake, you can internally boost your alkalinity thanks to your liver!
- Your pancreas thrives on alkalinity. Too much acid in your system throws off your pancreas. If you eat alkaline foods, your pancreas can regulate your blood sugars.

- Your kidneys also help to keep your body alkaline. When they are overwhelmed by an acidic diet, they cannot do their job

- The lymph fluids function most efficiently in an alkaline system. They remove acid waste. Acidic systems not only have a slower lymph flow causing acids to be stored; they can also cause acids to be reabsorbed through lymphatic ducts in your intestines that would typically be excreted.

MENTAL FOCUS

The alkalinity of the system is one of the best ways to focus and strengthen the mind. Just as the rest of the body is poorly affected by acid-forming foods and other toxins, so is your brain. And as we all know, it should be possible to control your emotions and decision making with your mind. Guess what? If your body is too acidic and is not alkaline, your mental clarity will be cloudy, your decision making could be off, as well as your emotional state.

DETOX

Another huge benefit of an alkaline lifestyle is detoxification. First, you are going to be cutting out processed foods that are continually adding toxins to your system.

Secondly, you are going to be eating foods that allow your body to detox and rid itself of the acids that have built up in your system all this time. When we detoxify our bodies, our emotions, bodily functions, and mental functions can operate at their optimum levels.

The number of benefits that come with living alkaline are numerous. As you help your body rebalance its optimal blood pH, you will find, as we did, that you have never felt better. We are still seeing improvement and reaping the rewards of this holistic approach to not only eating alkaline foods but living alkaline.

Alkaline vs. Acidic? Sounds like the title fight for a lightweight boxing match. In reality, it is a fight, a fight for the pH balance of your body. pH levels are basically the measure of how acidic a liquid is.

Our bodies function optimally when our blood is at about 7.35 - 7.45 pH.
pH levels range from 0 to 14. 0 is the highest level of acidity, but basically, everything 0-7 would be considered acidic. The 7-14 range is alkaline.

Before we dive into complicated pH discussions, here is one thing to understand:

-The alkaline <u>diet is not about changing or "raising" your pH</u>. This is where many alkaline guides go wrong. You see, our body is smart enough to **self-regulate** our pH for us, no matter what we eat. Unfortunately, when you constantly bombard your body with acid-forming foods (for example processed foods, fast food, alcohol, sugar, crappy carbs, and even too much meat) you torture your body with incredible stress. Why? Well because it has to work harder to maintain that optimal pH…

Here's simple example…

Imagine you immerse yourself in a bath filled with ice. You say, but hey, my body can self-regulate its optimal temperature, right? And yes, it can. But it will eventually collapse, and you will get ill. The same happens with nutrition and our blood pH.

You can spend years indulging in toxic, processed, acid-forming foods that only deprive your body of its vital nutrients, saying: "But hey, my body will self-regulate its optimal blood pH."

And again, it will...but sooner or later it will give up and manifest a disease. It will accumulate fat as its natural defense function to protect your body from over-acidity. We don't wanna end up there, right?

So, to sum up- the alkaline diet is a natural, holistic system, a nutritional lifestyle that advocates the consumption of fresh, unprocessed foods that are rich in nutrients. These are called alkaline foods, and they help your body stimulate its optimal healing functions. Yes! A healthy body needs nutrients, and fresh fruits and vegetables are great for that.

The problem is that nowadays, most diets are filled with acid-forming foods that eventually make it hard for the body to regulate its optimal, healthy blood pH. Acidosis is very common in this day and age thanks to things we drink as well: coffee, alcohol, sugar, crappy carbs, and sodas all have an acidic effect on our bodies. Not to mention the chemicals many people take in through things like smoking and drugs (even prescription drugs have this effect).

There are many ways that you could become acidic. Eating acid-forming foods, stress, taking in too many toxins, and bodily processes all cause acidity in the body. Our internal systems try to balance themselves out and bring pH up with the help of alkaline minerals that we can ingest through our diet. If we do not take in a higher percentage of alkaline than acidic foods, we can become too acidic.

When you are acidic, it makes every process that your body does typically much more difficult or impossible for it to accomplish. We cannot absorb the beneficial nutrients we need from our food correctly. Our cells are not able to produce energy efficiently. Our bodies are not able to fix damaged cells properly. We will not be able to detoxify properly. Fatigue and illness will drag you down. Sounds horrible; does it not? Here are some signs that you are overly acidic:

- ✓ Feeling tired all the time. You have no physical or mental drive at all.
- ✓ You always feel cold.
- ✓ You get sick easily.
- ✓ You are depressed or just feel "blah" all the time for no real reason
- ✓ You are easily overstimulated and stressed by noise, light, etc.
- ✓ You get headaches for no apparent reason
- ✓ You get watery eyes or inflamed eyelids.
- ✓ Your teeth are sensitive and may crack or chip

- ✓ Your gums are inflamed, and you are susceptible to canker sores
- ✓ You have recurring bouts with throat problems including tonsillitis
- ✓ Acidic stomach with acid indigestion and reflux is always an issue
- ✓ Your fingernails crack, split, and break
- ✓ You have super dry hair that sheds and is hay-like with split ends
- ✓ You have dry, ashy skin
- ✓ Your skin breaks out in acne or is irritated when you sweat
- ✓ You get leg cramps and spasms (this includes restless leg syndrome).

Changing your diet to one that is full of alkaline foods is one of the easiest and best things you can do for your overall health. I was so ecstatic that I did! And the best thing is- we will be combining alkaline foods with keto friendly meals to make it easy, delicious and fun! Much simpler to follow for the long term.

But the way we see it is this- it's perfect! Plus, it's not a diet, it's a lifestyle.

What I really like about the alkaline diet is that you don't have to be 100% perfect. It's enough to make sure you add a ton of greens and veggies and make your diet rich in alkaline foods.

It's easy to do when you focus on serving your lunch or dinner with a big green salad or start drinking alkaline keto smoothies and juices.

When it comes to the alkaline diet, there is something called the 70/30 rule meaning that about 70% of your diet should be fresh, nutrient dense alkaline-forming foods and the remaining 30% can be acid- forming foods (however they still should be clean and organic, for example, grass-fed meat or organic eggs).

The common mistakes with the ketogenic diets:
The most common mistake that people make is that they do not include enough veggies with their keto animal-based foods. That can cause imbalance and acidity. Hence, I am such a big fan of keto and alkaline diets combined together. Green vegetables are a fantastic addition to your keto diet.

They will help you have more energy and also add more variety to your diet. Alkaline Keto juicing is a simple to follow, natural tool to help you drink more vegetables. For many people, drinking veggies is actually easier than eating them.

The real keto lifestyle is about variety, abundance, and energy. It's hard to be successful with a keto diet if a menu consists entirely of animal products.

Combining Alkaline with Keto

As surprising as it may sound, the ketogenic diet is actually pretty close to the alkaline diet.

The primary common rule is:
Eat real food, eat clean food. Relax. Reduce stress. Enjoy the nature...

And these are the alkaline-keto guidelines to help you create vibrant health and energy:

-add a lot of greens (one of the best ways is through the alkaline keto juices)

-add lots of healthy fats like omega 3 and saturated fats (again, alkaline keto juices will help you do that too)

-eat fresh, unrefined, natural foods

-get rid of processed carbs

-reduce fruit that is high in sugar (the recipes contained in this book only use low sugar fruit, and other fruit is used very sparingly, in small amounts, just to taste)

-eliminate gluten and sugar-containing foods and drinks

-get rid of refined oils

-consume moderate healthy protein (alkaline diet focuses more on plant-based protein; however, some quality plant-based protein is also OK on this diet as long as you add in a ton of greens and veggies; similarly, while the keto diet is mostly known for recommending animal-based protein, plant-based protein from leafy greens, nuts and seeds is also keto-friendly).

The alkaline keto diet can be created in different versions. Listen to your body and give it what it needs to thrive.

Your Wellness Books Email Newsletter

Before we dive into the recipes, we would like to offer you free access to our VIP Wellness Newsletter.

www.yourwellnessbooks.com/newsletter

Here's what's in for you:

-healthy, clean food recipes and tips delivered to your email

-motivation and inspiration to help you stay on track

-discounts and giveaways

-notifications about our new books (at massively reduced prices)

-healthy eating resources to help you on your journey

No Fluff, no spam. Only helpful and easy to follow info!

Sign up link (copy this link to your phone, tablet, or PC):

Problems with signing up? Email us at

info@yourwellnessbooks.com

www.yourwellnessbooks.com/email-newsletter

About the Recipes-Measurements Used in the Recipes

The cup measurement I use is the American Cup measurement.
I also use it for dry ingredients. If you are new to it, let me help you:
If you don't have American Cup measures, just use a metric or
imperial liquid measuring jug and fill your jug with your ingredient
to the corresponding level. Here's how to go about it:

1 American Cup= 250ml= 8 Fl.oz.

For example:

If a recipe calls for 1 cup of almonds, simply place your almonds into
your measuring jug until it reaches the 250 ml/8oz marks.

I hope you found it helpful. I know that different countries use
different measurements, and I wanted to make things simple for
you. I have also noticed that very often those who are used to
American Cup measurements complain about metric
measurements and vice versa. However, if you apply what I have
just explained, you will find it easy to use both.

Alkaline Keto Juice Recipes to Help You Thrive!

The golden rule is- when juicing, focus on:

-all kinds of veggies and greens that can be juiced

-low sugar fruit (for example lemons, limes, pomegranates, grapefruits)

Tips for getting started with juicing:

- Prepare your house: Clean out the fridge and pantry and be sure it's stocked with tons of fresh and frozen produce.

- Begin by adding a handful or so of organic baby spinach into your juices, especially if you're new to green juices.

- Invest in a good juicer and set an intention (for example: "I can't wait to get started on this journey and to juice 3 times a week" – is a simple to follow through goal and intention).

- Prepare all your juices the night before and store them in air-tight containers for the following day. Making all the juices at once can save time in clean up and ensures you're ready with fresh juice whenever needed.

- There are so many variations of juicing, you can use the recipes and add or take away ingredients. Feel free to swap for your favorite ingredients, just make sure you're getting a tasty variety throughout the day.

The juicer I like to use is Omega Juicer. However, any other cold pressed juicer will do.

You can learn more about the recommended tools and resources at:

www.YourWellnessBooks.com/resources

Make sure you wash all the ingredients before you proceed to your juicing rituals.

Now, it's time for the recipes. I am so excited for you!

Avocado Oil Green Juice for Energy & Weight Loss

Avocado oil offers good fat to help you absorb the minerals and vitamins from the juice. I love this juice whenever I need "an injection of energy." Himalaya salt adds alkaline minerals and makes this juice taste amazing. If you like spicy juices, feel free to add in some hot sauce, or chili powder.

Servings: 2

Ingredients:

- 1 lemon, peeled
- 1 lime, peeled
- 2 celery stalks, chopped
- a handful of arugula leaves
- 2 big cucumbers, peeled and chopped
- 2 tablespoons avocado oil
- Himalayan salt to taste
- Optional: A couple dashes of hot habanero sauce or chili powder

Instructions:

1. Place through a juicer.
2. Juice and combine with the avocado oil and Himalayan salt.
3. Serve in a glass and enjoy!

No More Sugar Cravings Juice

This green juice recipe is beginner friendly, and it's also designed to help you fight sugar cravings.

The creamy consistency of this juice, micronutrients from green juice and super healthy fats from coconut oil will help you say no to sugar. Ginger adds anti-inflammatory properties.

Serves: 2

Ingredients:

- 1 cup spinach leaves
- 2-inch ginger, peeled
- 2 tablespoons melted coconut oil
- 1 cup of thick coconut milk
- Half teaspoon Ashwagandha
- Optional: stevia to sweeten

Instructions:

1. Place the spinach and ginger through a juicer.
2. Extract the juice, pour it in a big glass.
3. Combine with coconut milk and oil.
4. Add in the Ashwagandha.
5. Stir well and enjoy.

Beautiful Skin Juice

This recipe is delicious and helpful for those who don't enjoy juicing greens. It also uses turmeric that is very alkalizing and also offers anti-inflammatory benefits.

When peeling, cutting and juicing turmeric, I recommend you use gloves (unless you want to walk around with orange nails and hands for the next 2 days lol).

Servings: 2

Ingredients:

- 2 big red bell peppers, chopped
- 1 big yellow bell pepper
- 2 inches of turmeric, peeled (use gloves)
- 2 lemons
- 2 tablespoons flax seed oil

Instructions:

1. Juice all the ingredients using a juicer.
2. Add in the flax seed oil.
3. Serve in a glass.
4. Enjoy!

Lemon Digestion and Weight Loss Tonic

This recipe helps maintain a healthy digestive system and stimulate weight loss (thanks to grapefruits). It also makes your water taste great!

Servings: 2

Ingredients:

- 1 cup of mint leaves, chopped
- 1 grapefruit, peeled and chopped
- 1 lemon, peeled and halved
- 1 inch of ginger, peeled
- 1 cup of water
- Optional: stevia to sweeten

Instructions:

1. Place all the ingredients in a juicer. Juice.
2. Mix with water.
3. Serve chilled with some ice cubes.
4. Enjoy!

Super Hydrating Weight Loss Juice

This simple recipe is another easy to follow option for those who don't enjoy juicing leafy greens. Cucumbers taste really delicious in juices and combine really well with coconut oil and milk.

Servings: 2

Ingredients:

- 4 big cucumbers, peeled and chopped
- 1 lime peeled and chopped
- 2 green bell peppers
- 2 tablespoons coconut oil, melted
- Himalaya salt to taste, if needed
- Half cup thick coconut milk

Instructions:

1. Place all the ingredients through a juicer.
2. Extract the juice.
3. Pour into a chilled glass.
4. Add in the coconut oil and coconut milk.
5. Taste with Himalaya salt if needed.
6. Enjoy!

Soft Balance Green Juice

Celery juice offers anti-inflammatory properties and Vitamin C to help you enjoy more energy and take care of your immune system. Maca powder is a fantastic hormone balancer, and I love using it with this juice. Red bell pepper makes it taste really delicious, and so does the cinnamon and nutmeg powder.

Servings: 2

Ingredients:

- 1 cup celery, chopped
- 1 inch of ginger, peeled
- 1 red bell pepper
- 2 tablespoons avocado oil
- half teaspoon cinnamon powder
- half teaspoon maca powder
- cinnamon and nutmeg powder to taste

Instructions:

1. Juice all the ingredients using a juicer.
2. Pour in a glass.
3. Add in the avocado oil, maca, cinnamon, and nutmeg powder.
4. Stir well, serve and enjoy!

On the Go Alkaline Keto Juice Shot (Liver Lover)

This recipe is perfect if you are too busy to juice…

You know…setting up the juicer, cleaning up.

Well, this recipe doesn't even need a proper juicer. A simple lemon squeezer will do.

This simple recipe helps detoxify the liver, it works really well first thing in the morning.

Serves: 1

Ingredients:

- 2 lemons
- 1 tablespoon avocado oil or olive oil
- Pinch of Himalaya salt

Instructions:

1. Juice the lemons.
2. In a small glass, combine the lemon juice with the oil and Himalaya salt.
3. Stir well, say 3-2-1 and drink.
4. To your health!

(yea…sometimes it's about the taste, and sometimes it's about the benefit)

Energy Replenishment Juice

This recipe uses coconut water to help you spice up your green juice and make it taste amazing.

Serves: 1-2

Ingredients:

- 1 cup of coconut water
- 1 cup spinach leaves
- 1-inch ginger
- 1 grapefruit
- Ice cubes

Instructions:

1. Juice the spinach, ginger, and grapefruit.
2. Combine with coconut water and ice cubes.
3. Serve and enjoy!

Red Cabbage Detox Juice

Cabbage is an excellent source of sulfur, which helps purify the blood and detoxify the liver. Fennel and mint help create a nice flavor while adding in more healing nutrients to help you thrive.

Servings: 2

Ingredients:

- 1 small red cabbage
- 1 fennel bulb
- A handful of mint leaves
- Half cup almond milk
- 2 tablespoons melted coconut oil
- Optional- stevia to sweeten

Procedure:

1. Juice all the ingredients.
2. Add the almond milk and coconut oil.
3. Stir well.
4. Enjoy!

Vitamin C Green Juice for Natural Energy & Weight Loss

This simple juice recipe offers a fantastic combination of greens with alkaline keto friendly fruits and healthy fats. It will help you feel energized while eliminating sugar cravings.

Servings: 1-2

Ingredients:

- 2 grapefruits, peeled
- 1 cup kale leaves, chopped
- 1-inch ginger
- 2 tablespoon flax seed oil or sesame oil
- Optional: stevia to sweeten

Instructions:

1. Juice the grapefruits, kale leaves, and ginger.
2. Combine with flax seed oil (or sesame oil).
3. If needed, sweeten with stevia.
4. Serve and enjoy!

Light Alkaline Keto Juice

This juice is particularly useful for healthy eyesight and beautiful skin as it is packed with Vitamins A and C.

It also helps fight inflammation and takes care of your liver.

Ingredients:

- 1 cup radish, cut into smaller pieces
- 1-inch ginger
- 1 lime, peeled
- 1 fennel bulb, cut into smaller pieces
- 1 tablespoon sesame or flax seed oil
- Pinch of Himalayan salt

Instructions:

1. Juice the radish, ginger, lime, and fennel.
2. Add in the Himalayan salt and oil.
3. Stir well, serve and enjoy!

Apple Cider Antioxidant Juice for Optimal Energy

This recipe is full of miraculous nutrients to help you get rid of toxins. Its therapeutic properties are enhanced by Apple Cider Vinegar.

Servings: 1-2

Ingredients:

- 2 cucumbers, peeled and sliced
- Half cup of parsley leaves
- Half cup of mint leaves
- 2 tablespoons of olive oil
- 1 tablespoon apple cider vinegar (organic)
- Himalayan salt to taste (optional)

Instructions:

1. Juice all the ingredients.
2. Add in the olive oil, apple cider vinegar, Himalayan salt, and black pepper.
3. Serve and enjoy!

***To learn more about Apple Cider Vinegar (for health, home, and beauty), I highly recommend you read my book:

Apple Cider Vinegar: The Miraculous Natural Remedy!: Holistic Solutions & Proven Healing Recipes for Health, Beauty, and Home

If your goal is weight loss and body detoxification, you can start adding about 1-2 tablespoons (a day) of quality, organic, apple cider vinegar to your alkaline-keto drinks.

Apple cider vinegar goes really well with therapeutic alkaline keto juices (and also smoothies). It's inexpensive and very effective.

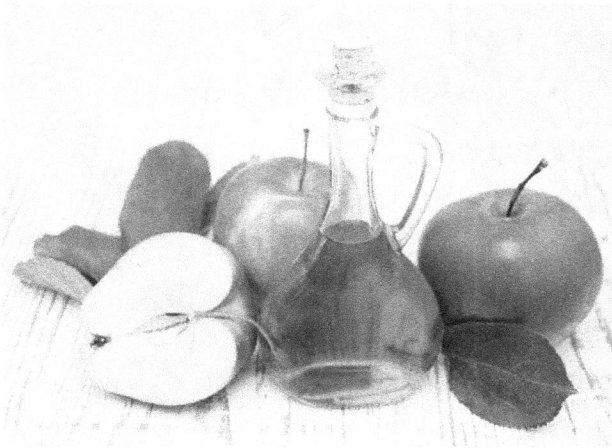

Fat Burn Weight Loss Herbal Alkaline Keto Juice

This recipe fuses the low sugar alkaline fruits with horsetail infusion. Horsetail infusion is an excellent natural remedy to get rid of water retention, lose weight, and burn fat. It's full of alkaline minerals and blends really well with this juice.

Ingredients:

- A handful of fresh mint leaves
- 1 grapefruit, peeled
- 1 lime, peeled
- Half inch ginger, peeled
- 2 cucumbers, peeled
- Half cup horsetail infusion cooled down
- Optional: stevia to sweeten

Instructions:

1. First, juice all the ingredients.
2. Combine with horsetail infusion. Add stevia if needed.
3. Serve and enjoy!

No More Insomnia Alkaline Keto Juice

This delicious herbal juice uses verbena- a herb used to stimulate relaxation and peace of mind.

Servings: 1-2

Ingredients:

- 1 cup verbena infusion, cooled down a bit (use 1 teabag per cup)
- 2 grapefruits, peeled and sliced
- 1 cup chopped celery
- A handful of fresh mint leaves
- Stevia to sweeten

Procedure:

1. Juice the grapefruits, celery, and mint leaves.
2. Mix the juice with the infusion.
3. Stir well and add stevia for naturally sweet taste.
4. Enjoy!

Verbena is a pretty safe herb, but there is not enough information to confirm whether it can be used during pregnancy or breastfeeding. The same applies to possible contraindications with other medications. I always recommend consulting with your doctor first.

Pomegranate Avocado Anti-Sugar Cravings Juice

This recipe will help you get rid of sugar cravings while feeding your body with a myriad of nutrients it needs to thrive. Pomegranate juice is full of alkaline minerals as well as Vitamin C.

It's a natural antioxidant and anti-inflammatory. It blends really well with ginger, turmeric, and mint. You can't juice avocado...but you can use avocado oil.

Servings: 2

Ingredients:

- 1 cup pomegranate seeds
- 1-inch ginger root, peeled
- 1-inch turmeric root, peeled
- A handful of fresh mint leaves
- 2 tablespoons of avocado oil
- Stevia to sweeten (optional)

Procedure:

1. Juice the pomegranate seeds, ginger, turmeric, and mint.
2. Combine with avocado oil.
3. Serve and enjoy!

Alkalizing Mojito Juice

It's time for a simple and super healthy, non-alcoholic version of mojito!

Servings: 2-3

Ingredients:

- 1 cucumber, peeled and sliced
- Half cup fresh mint leaves
- 2 limes, peeled and sliced
- A few mint leaves to garnish
- A few lime slices to garnish
- 3 cups alkaline (or filtered) water
- Stevia to sweeten (optional)

Instructions:

1. Juice all the ingredients (except the mint and lime slices for garnishing)
2. Pour the fresh juice into a tall water jar or pitcher.
3. Add fresh water and ice cubes.
4. Now, add the mint leaves and lime slices.
5. Stir in well, chill in a fridge for a few hours, and serve.
6. Enjoy!

Cucumber Kale Weight Loss Juice

While it's hard to eat a mountain of greens and cucumbers, it's easy to drink their juice and get all the vital nutrients from them. Avocado oil offers good fat to help you absorb the minerals and vitamins from the juice.

Servings: 2

Ingredients:

- 1 cup of kale, chopped
- 4 big cucumbers, peeled and chopped
- 2 limes, peeled
- 2 tablespoons of avocado oil
- Himalaya salt and black pepper to taste (optional)

Instructions:

1. Place through a juicer.
2. Pour into a glass and mix in some Himalayan salt and black pepper to taste. Stir in the avocado oil.
3. Enjoy!

Super Tasty Spinach Juice (Not Kidding!)

While pure spinach juice can be a bit hardcore, this recipe is a bit different as it uses coconut milk and delicious spices...It's very nutritious and rich in good fats. And yes...you still get all the benefits of drinking green juice...

Serves: 2

Ingredients:

- 2 cups of fresh spinach leaves
- 2-inch ginger, peeled
- 1 cup almond milk, unsweetened
- 1 cup coconut milk, unsweetened
- 2 tablespoons coconut oil
- 1 teaspoon cinnamon powder
- Pinch of nutmeg powder
- Optional: stevia to sweeten

Instructions:

1. Place all the ingredients through a juicer.
2. Extract the juice, pour it in a big glass.
3. Add in some melted coconut oil, coconut and almond milk as well as spices and stevia.
4. Stir well and enjoy.

Tomato Mediterranean Antioxidant Juice

Tomato, ginger, and good oils make an excellent combination. Mediterranean spices take it to the next level!

Servings: 2

Ingredients:

- 8 big organic tomatoes, chopped
- 2 inches of ginger, peeled
- 2 garlic cloves, peeled
- 2 tablespoons olive oil
- 2 tablespoons Mediterranean spices (oregano, thyme, rosemary- it's really up to you)
- Himalaya salt to taste

Instructions:

1. Juice all the ingredients using a juicer.
2. Combine with olive oil and spices.
3. Enjoy!

Simple Flavored Kale Juice

While I definitely don't promote the idea of juicing sugary fruits, it's absolutely fine to add a bit of apple to your green juice to make it taste sweeter.

Servings: 2

Ingredients:

- 2 cups of kale, chopped
- 1 green apple, peeled and chopped
- 1 lemon, peeled and halved
- 1 inch of ginger, peeled
- 1-inch turmeric, peeled
- 1 tablespoon flaxseed oil
- 1 teaspoon cinnamon powder
- 1 teaspoon maca powder
- Optional: stevia to sweeten

Instructions:

1. Place all the ingredients in a juicer.
2. Juice, mix with flaxseed oil, maca, and cinnamon powder.
3. Serve in a glass.
4. If needed, sweeten with stevia.
5. Enjoy!

Easy Light Green Juice

This is a super hydrating, alkalizing green juice with a nice, light flavor.

Servings: 2

Ingredients:

- 4 medium cucumbers, peeled and chopped
- 1 romaine lettuce
- 2 limes
- 2 tablespoons avocado oil
- Optional: Himalayan salt to taste

Instructions:

1. Place all the ingredients through a juicer.
2. Extract the juice.
3. Mix with avocado oil and Himalayan salt
4. Pour into a chilled glass and enjoy!

Naturally Sweet Celery Juice

Red bell peppers are one of my favorite veggies to juice.
They are naturally sweet and full of vitamins and minerals. They make any green juice taste amazing. This recipe is perfect for people who are just getting started on juicing celery and want to make a juice that feels nice.

Servings: 2

Ingredients:

- 1 cup celery, chopped
- 3 red bell peppers, chopped
- 1 inch of ginger, peeled
- 1 lime, peeled
- 1 cup water, filtered, preferably alkaline
- Mint leaves to garnish
- Optional: stevia to sweeten if needed

Instructions:

1. Juice all the ingredients using a juicer.
2. Pour in a big glass or a jar. Combine with water.
3. Stir well. Sweeten with stevia if needed.
4. Garnish with mint leaves.
5. Serve and enjoy!

Coconut Kale Energy Boosting Concoction

Compared to other juicing recipes, this one is relatively simple and quick to make as it leverages the coconut water. Just perfect as a quick, energy-boosting juice. Great for those who are just getting started on green juice! Apple cider vinegar is an added bonus.

Servings: 2

Ingredients:

- 1 cup kale, chopped
- Half of green apple, peeled and chopped
- 1 cup of coconut water, unsweetened
- 1 tablespoon coconut oil
- 1 tablespoon apple cider vinegar
- 1 teaspoon cinnamon powder

Instructions:

1. Juice the kale and apple.
2. Pour into a glass and mix with 1 cup of coconut water.
3. Stir well, add in 1 teaspoon of cinnamon powder.
4. Stir again and add the coconut oil and apple cider vinegar.
5. Stir well again, serve and enjoy!

Simple Chlorophyll Juice

This juice is great for boosting your energy and stimulating weight loss. Liquid chlorophyll is a fantastic way of enriching your juice with more nutrients, and it's perfect if you are too busy to juice the heaps of greens. To make this recipe, you don't even need an Omega Juicer, you could easily do with a simple lemon squeezer. If you are looking for liquid chlorophyll, or green powder recommendation, please check our website: www.YourWellnessBooks.com/resources

Servings: 2

Ingredients:

- 2 big grapefruits
- 1 cup thick coconut milk, full fat, unsweetened
- 1 tablespoon avocado oil
- Half teaspoon cinnamon powder
- A few drops of liquid chlorophyll
- Stevia to sweeten- optional

Instructions:

1. Juice the grapefruits (a lemon squeezer tool like the one on the picture below, will do for this recipe).

2. Combine the juice with avocado oil, coconut milk, cinnamon powder, and liquid chlorophyll.

3. Stir well, serve in a glass and enjoy!

A simple lemon squeezer tool like this one can be a real life-saver. Perfect for simple juice recipes including limes, lemons, and grapefruits (healthy alkaline keto fruits!).

Simple to use and inexpensive! Be sure to purchase a lemon squeezer tool that is sharp enough to juice grapefruits as well. Easy peasy lemon squeezy!

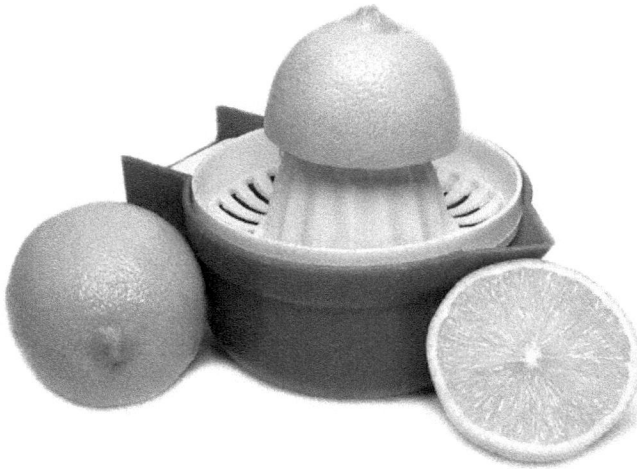

Green Tea Bullet Proof Vitamin C Juice

This recipe uses green tea to help you boost your energy levels and burn fat. Ginger adds to anti-inflammatory properties. Then, there is grapefruit, super-rich in Vitamin C and alkaline minerals.

That mix combines really well with coconut oil. So tasty and good for you! Once again, for this recipe, you don't even need a fancy juicer. A simple lemon squeezer will do.

Servings: 2

Ingredients:

- 1 big grapefruit
- 1-inch ginger, peeled
- 1 cup green tea, cooled down (use 1 teabag per cup)
- 2 tablespoons coconut oil
- Stevia to sweeten if needed

Instructions:

1. Make the green tea, add in ginger, and leave covered to boil.
2. In the meantime, juice grapefruit using a lemon squeezer or a juicer.
3. In a small hand blender, combine the grapefruit juice and coconut oil. Process until smooth.

4. Once the green tea cools down, pour the juice into a big glass or a jar, and combine with the tea. Serve as it is or chilled. Enjoy!

Grapefruit juice benefits:

-helps in weight loss (it's low in calories and high in nutrients)

-very low in carbs and sugars

-stimulates the lymphatic system, helping you feel lighter and more energized

-boost the immune system

-Very alkalizing!

Beta Carotene Powerhouse for Healthy-Looking Skin

This juice is a fantastic combination of tomatoes, turmeric, and ginger to help you have beautiful and healthy-looking skin while enjoying more energy without having to rely on caffeine.

Servings: 2

Ingredients:

- 6 big tomatoes, chopped
- 2-inch turmeric, peeled
- 2-inch ginger, peeled
- 2 tablespoons olive oil
- Pinch of Himalayan salt

Instructions:

1. Juice all the ingredients.
2. Pour into a glass and add in the olive oil and Himalayan salt.
3. Enjoy!

A Restorative Antioxidant Non-Green Juice

This juice shows once again that healthy juicing can go beyond juicing greens. Tomatoes blend very well with grapefruits and ginger.

Servings: 2

Ingredients:

- 4 tomatoes, cut into smaller pieces
- 1-inch ginger, peeled
- 2 big grapefruits, peeled and cut into smaller pieces
- 2 tablespoons avocado oil

Instructions:

1. Juice all the ingredients.
2. Combine with avocado oil.
3. Serve in a big glass and enjoy!

Veggie Lover Juice

Elena? Why juicing? Why not just eat those veggies?

My mom used to ask me this question all the time.

Well....would it be even possible to eat through a massive pile of veggies below? Juicing makes it easier. Think of all the micronutrients your body is getting in an easy to absorb "vitamin and mineral injection".

Servings: 4

Ingredients:

- 3 medium carrots, peeled and cut into smaller pieces
- 1 beet (with greens), peeled
- 4 large tomatoes, cut into smaller pieces
- 2 large handfuls spinach
- Half head cabbage, chopped
- 1 red bell pepper, chopped
- 1 large celery stalk, chopped
- A handful of mint leaves
- 4 tablespoons avocado oil

Instructions:

1. Juice all the ingredients.
2. Pour into a big jar, combine with avocado oil, serve in smaller glasses and enjoy!
3. If needed, season with some Himalaya salt.

Suggestions- this recipe is perfect for big batch juicing.

It will help you restore balance and energy.

You can use your juicing time to feed your mind and body with positive information or music.

If you're looking for wellness audiobooks to keep you company on your juicing journey, we warmly invite you to check out our collection:

www.YourWellnessBooks.com/audiobooks

Delicious Color Juice

While pure green juice might be a bit too "hardcore" even for experienced juicing fanatics, it tastes amazing when mixed with other ingredients, such as red bell peppers. The color is amazing too!

Servings: 2

Ingredients:

- Half cabbage, chopped
- 4 red bell peppers, sliced
- 2 limes, peeled
- 2 tablespoons avocado oil

Instructions:

1. Juice all the ingredients.
2. Pour into a glass and mix with some avocado oil.
3. Enjoy!

Mixed Green Juice

This recipe is great if you happen to have some arugula leaves leftovers and don't feel like going for another salad. And yes, arugula juice tastes amazing when mixed with other ingredients!

Servings: 2

Ingredients:

- 1 cup arugula leaves
- A few slices of green apple
- 1 lemon, peeled and cut into smaller pieces
- 1 tablespoon avocado oil

Instructions:

1. Place though a juicer.
2. Juice and pour into a glass or a small jar.
3. Stir in some avocado oil.
4. Enjoy!

Sexy Aphrodisiac Green Juice

Once again, we are juicing arugula leaves while adding in some sweetness from red bell peppers and flavors from cilantro and mint. Arugula is a super nourishing and hydrating leafy green. It's recommended for bone health and it also helps reduce inflammation in the body. Och…and it's an aphrodisiac too!

Servings: 2

Ingredients:

- 1 cup arugula leaves
- 2 red bell peppers, chopped
- 2 tablespoons fresh cilantro leaves
- 2 tablespoons fresh mint leaves
- 2 tablespoons avocado oil

Instructions:

1. Place all the ingredients though a juicer.
2. Juice and add in the avocado oil.
3. Serve and enjoy!

Healing Ashwagandha Juice

Ashwagandha powder is a great choice to help you re-balance your energy levels while feeling more relaxed. Coconut milk makes this juice creamy and soft.

Servings: 2

Ingredients:

- 2 red bell peppers, chopped
- 1 lime, peeled and chopped
- 1 cup coconut milk
- 2 tablespoons coconut oil
- Half teaspoon Ashwagandha powder

Instructions:

1. Juice the bell peppers and a lime.
2. Pour into a small hand blender and combine with coconut milk, coconut oil and Ashwagandha.
3. Blend until smooth and creamy.
4. Pour into a glass and enjoy!

Mint Parsley Delight

Parsley leaves add in a ton of vitamins and nutrients such as Vitamin A, Vitamin C and Iron. Mint helps in digestion and brings an amazing aroma to the table. Almond milk makes this juice even more nutritious (and creamy)!

Servings: 2

Ingredients:

- A handful of fresh mint leaves
- A handful of fresh parsley leaves
- 2 lemons, peeled and chopped
- 1 cup almond milk
- Stevia to sweeten, if needed
- 2 tablespoons avocado oil

Instructions:

1. Juice mint and parsley.
2. Pour into a glass or a small jar.
3. Add the almond milk, stevia and avocado oil.
4. Stir well and enjoy!

Creamy Turmeric Drink

Turmeric is full of polyphenols that help well in weight loss.

It's a great addition to your juices and creates a nice, spicy aroma that is very easy to get hooked on.

I love combining this juice with full-fat, creamy coconut milk and cinnamon. So yummy, healthy, alkaline and keto!

Servings: 2-3

Ingredients:

- 3-inch turmeric, peeled
- 4 cucumbers, peeled and chopped
- 1 cup warm coconut milk
- 1 tablespoon coconut oil
- 1 teaspoon cinnamon

Instructions:

1. Heat up the coconut milk and add in the cinnamon and coconut oil.
2. Stir well and set aside.
3. In the meantime, juice the cucumbers and turmeric.
4. Add the fresh juice to the coconut milk concoction.
5. Stir well, serve and enjoy!

Lime Mint Alkaline Water

This recipe uses fresh juice to make your water taste delicious!

Servings: 3-4

Ingredients:

- ¼ cup mint leaves, fresh
- 2 limes, peeled and chopped
- 4-inch ginger, peeled
- 4 big cucumbers, peeled and chopped
- 4 cups water, filtered, preferably alkaline
- Optional: stevia to sweeten if desired

Instructions:

1. Place the mint leaves, limes, ginger and cucumbers through a juicer.
2. Juice.
3. Pour into a big water jar and combine with 4 cups of filtered water.
4. Stir well, if needed sweeten with stevia.
5. Enjoy!

Pomegranate Green Juice

With pomegranate, you are sure to enjoy a juice that is full of antioxidants and nutrients that are good for weight loss.

Oh, and we are sneaking in some greens too. Great way to make use of some salad leftovers! Some days, I really like to keep it simple.

Servings: 2

Ingredients:

- 1 cup pomegranate seeds
- 1 cup of mixed greens of your choice
- 2 tablespoons flaxseed oil

Instructions:

1. Juice the greens and pomegranates.
2. Pour into a glass and stir in the flaxseed oil.
3. Serve and enjoy!

Coconut Flavored Veggie Juice

The juice ingredients are rich in phytonutrients and antioxidants. Coconut oil makes this concoction taste really delicious, while helping you reduce sugar and carb cravings too.

Focus on adding greens and good oils and it will be so much easier to live a healthy lifestyle! This recipe proves just that.

Servings: 2

Ingredients:

- 1 cup kale, chopped
- 3 carrots, peeled
- 2 tablespoons coconut oil, melted
- 1 cup thick coconut milk
- Half teaspoon cinnamon powder to serve

Instructions:

1. Place the kale and carrots through a juicer.
2. Juice and pour into a glass.
3. Stir in the coconut oil and coconut milk.
4. Sprinkle over a bit of cinnamon powder.
5. Serve and enjoy!

Bonus Recipe – Gluten-Free Pancakes Made with the Pulp

You can use the pulp from your juices to make healthy, low-carb, gluten-free pancakes. The recipe below is a template that you can personalize depending on your taste preferences.

You can make sweet pancakes using stevia and using pulp from limes, lemons or pomegranates.

Vegetable pulp works better for spicy or savory pancakes.

Ingredients:

- 4 tablespoons pulp
- 1 teaspoon spices (depending on your taste preferences)
- 2 organic eggs
- 8 tablespoons almond flour
- 1 tablespoon coconut oil (for the mixture)
- 3 tablespoons coconut oil (for frying)

Instructions:

1. Heat up the coconut oil in a skillet (medium heat).
2. In the meantime, blend the pulp, eggs, flour and 1 tablespoon coconut oil, until smooth creamy mixture.
3. Form little pancakes and start frying on both sides.
4. Serve and enjoy!

Let's finish this book with a few words of motivation and inspiration.

It's all about taking meaningful and inspired action.

Ditch perfection for progress. Focus on daily micro steps. Healthy choices. Ask yourself- is this taking me closer to my goals?

Cultivate positive self-talk. Stop beating yourself up.

Beautiful results will start taking place.

Think where you will be 5 years from now...The baby steps will compound into a big transformation.

Be patient. Focus on the here and now.

Thank you again for reading.

I am really grateful for you,

Until next time,

Wishing you all the best on your journey,

Elena

www.amazon.com/author/elenagarcia

We Need Your Help

One more thing, before you go, could you please do us a quick favor?

It would be great if you could leave us a short review online.

Don't worry, it doesn't have to be long. One sentence is enough.

Let others know your favorite recipes and who you think this book can help.

Way too many people drink "normal" juices and don't even realize they are overdoing sugar...No wonder they give up...

Your review can inspire more and more people to learn the right method of juicing, that they can finally achieve their wellness and weight loss goals the way they deserve.

Your honest review is critical.

Thank You for your support!

Join Our VIP Readers' Newsletter to Boost Your Wellbeing

Would you like to be notified about our new health and wellness books?

How about receiving them at deeply discounted prices? And before anyone else?

What about awesome giveaways, latest health tips, and motivation?

If that is something you are interested in, please visit the link below to join our newsletter:

www.yourwellnessbooks.com/email-newsletter

It's 100% free + spam free (we hate spam as much as you do)

We promise we will only email you with valuable and relevant information, delicious recipes, and tips to help you on your journey.

Sign up link:

www.yourwellnessbooks.com/email-newsletter

More Wellness Books & Resources

Available at:

www.yourwellnessbooks.com

Final Words

Content Disclaimer

The information contained in this book is for informational and educational purposes only.

It is not an attempt by the writers or publisher to diagnose or prescribe, nor should it be construed to be such.

Readers are hereby encouraged to consult with a licensed health care professional concerning the information presented, which has been received from sources deemed reliable, but no guarantees, expressed or implied, can be made regarding the accuracy of same.

Therefore, readers are also encouraged to verify for themselves and to their own satisfaction the accuracy of all reports, recommendations, conclusions, comments, opinions, or anything else published herein before making any kind of decisions based upon what they have read.

If you have a medical condition, please consult your medical practitioner.

www.ingramcontent.com/pod-product-compliance
Lightning Source LLC
Chambersburg PA
CBHW071117030426
42336CB00013BA/2130